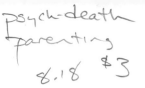

Empty Arms

Coping after miscarriage,
stillbirth and infant death

Sherokee Ilse

Edited by
Arlene Appelbaum

To help you accept, yet not forget.

ACKNOWLEDGMENTS

My sincere thanks and deep appreciation to:

My husband David, who shared his sorrow, strength and love with me.

Arlene Appelbaum, my editor, friend and firm supporter who kept me on track and gave me inspiration to continue.

The many midwives, doctors, nurses, clergy, bereaved parents, counselors, therapists and friends who read my manuscript at various stages, made helpful suggestions and emphasized the importance of this project.

My family and friends who remained lovingly interested and enthusiastic throughout my preoccupation with this book.

Graphic and design by David Fritz,
Barshuhn Design and AJ/Artifactory, Inc.

Copyright©1982 by Sherokee L. Ilse
3rd printing, 1985

For additional copies write to:
Sherokee Ilse
Box 165
Long Lake, MN 55356

Bulk rate available.

ISBN 0-9609456-4-4

For
BRENNAN WILLIAM ILSE

This is in memory of you . . . and all the other sons
and daughters who were so loved and wanted, but
did not live.

*On November 2, 1981, one day past our baby's due date, we were
told the most heartbreaking news parents can hear: "I'm sorry.
Your baby has died. There is no heartbeat."*

*Four long and grueling hours later we delivered a beautiful, peaceful
boy. Our son, Brennan, never took a breath, nor greeted the world
with a bellow. But he lived. And he will continue to live in our hearts
and memories always.*

*We hope that by sharing our experience, and what we have learned,
we can make it less painful for other parents and loved ones who
experience this tragedy . . . those who are left with empty arms.*

Fondly,

Sherokee & David

Sherokee and David Ilse

CONTENTS

For page numbers of specific topics and decisions, see index in the back of the book (page 55).

INTRODUCTION

Our hearts are broken. Our world seems like it has ended.
Our dreams, our hopes and our future with this child are over.
Our precious baby has died.

Babies are not supposed to die. Not your baby and not ours. But they do die. It has happened, and you are not prepared for this. You most likely are in shock and might wonder why it had to come to an end like this, because you probably loved and wanted this baby very much.

Many questions and fears are apt to arise in all of this confusion. Some of these questions might include: What will we do now? Will this nightmare end? Who do we tell and how? How will we make all of the decisions that we are so unprepared to make? No doubt you feel overwhelmed, all alone in your shock and grief and unprepared to cope. Grief is a very lonely process. You must work through it on your own, but you need not be alone. Others can help you, even as they grieve themselves.

Because I have lived through the loss of my son, I think I know how alone and empty you probably feel. I am deeply sorry your baby has died. I encourage you to make decisions that are right for you, just as David and I had to do. I know there is no right or best way to cope with your baby's death, but with this book I hope I can help lessen your pain, assist you in making decisions and speed your recovery.

The beginning of this book deals with specifics of your baby's death, whether it was due to a miscarriage, stillbirth or neonatal death. The main portion of it is written to help you cope with the decisions and concerns you might have in the days, weeks and

1

months to come and to begin recovering. You might want to read only the sections that pertain to your present needs and save the rest of the book until a later time. Do not allow the many sections to overwhelm you; take a section at a time if need be. My personal comments are included to help you feel less isolated and alone.

I hope you also will share this book with others, so that they can begin to understand what you are going through and what you might need.

David and I struggled, survived and grew from the painful experience of our son's death. So have others. I feel confident you can do it, too. I wish you the best as you work through this and recover.

LEARNING ABOUT YOUR BABY'S DEATH

When parents experience the unexpected death of their baby, it is natural for them to be unprepared, in shock and feeling a wide range of emotions from disbelief to anger to intense sorrow. Whether your baby died recently or awhile ago, you probably felt very devastated and confused. There is a profound sense of disappointment and loss when a baby dies. Your plans for bringing this baby home and the changes you were prepared to make have been thwarted. Your dreams, hopes and future with this child no longer can come true.

Whatever the circumstances of your baby's death, you probably will feel a strong sense of loss, sadness and maybe some bitterness at the unfairness of this tragedy. If you knew you were pregnant (whether it was full term or only months), or delivered a live baby who did not live long, you have come to know him or her as a special person in your life. Take time to think about what your baby meant to you and how you are feeling now. You will have many decisions to make; give yourself permission to do what is best for you. How you handle this loss will be different from how someone else does. You will experience some degree of grief, and what is crucial is how you accept your baby's death and work through that grief.

Mom, you have the added burden of the physical discomfort or complications from the miscarriage or the birth. This will make the next few hours, days and weeks even more stressful. Even so, you will need to grieve. Dad, you might be overlooked during this time and probably expected to be a pillar of strength while helping mom make it through all of this. Your feelings are important, and you also will need to grieve. You both have lost a precious child, someone you created together. You will be alone in your grief, yet you can share your sorrow and grow together.

When David and I were told that I would deliver a baby who was not alive, we didn't want to believe it and felt so confused. We kept hoping that it was a mistake and that it really wasn't true, because only four days earlier we had heard a strong heartbeat. It all seemed so unreal, so unfair. We had already experienced a miscarriage and certainly something like that couldn't happen to us again. We had been ready this time and were so sure that everything would go well. We had done everything right, and the love we felt for our child was so deep. Yet we had to accept that our wish for a healthy baby wouldn't come true.

MISCARRIAGE

A miscarriage can be a very lonely, confusing and sad experience, not just for you, but for those who come in contact with you. It is a sudden, unexpected and shocking loss of life that can shatter your plans and hopes for children, while your future might become clouded with doubt and anxiety.

A miscarriage is defined as delivery of a fetus prematurely before the twentieth week and before it can live on its own. Most miscarriages occur early in pregnancy, usually between the seventh and the fourteenth week. Statistics put the number of miscarriages at approximately 15 to 25 percent of all conceptions.

Most mothers are not admitted to the hospital, depending upon the length of the pregnancy and the individual circumstances. They are seen in clinics, doctors' offices and emergency rooms most often. Medical and emotional support is given at the time and at the two-week checkup. After that it is usually up to the couple to handle their emotional needs.

Many people who have not experienced it do not consider a miscarriage as the death of a baby, but rather as a fairly common occurrence and the end of a pregnancy. The messages parents often receive are to downplay what happened, get on with life and forget about it. These messages usually are given to minimize the parents' pain. Because you know you have lost your baby, and yet you hear conflicting reactions from others, you might be asking yourself the following question.

It was "only" a miscarriage. Why do I feel so upset and disappointed?

Even though the baby might not have been "visible," or perhaps people had not yet been informed, you still might experience feelings of disappointment, sadness or anger. You were expecting a baby and now you are not. The range of emotions and reactions vary drastically between people. Some might have been excited to be pregnant, while others did not particularly want to be pregnant at the time. Your needs, feelings and level of disappointment are unique.

It was not "just" a miscarriage; it was the death of your baby. Allow yourself to grieve and to say goodbye. Let others know how you feel and what you need. Discuss the plans, dreams and fantasies you had for your family and this baby. Find out how your partner feels and talk with other people who have experienced this.

I had a miscarriage, at two-and-a-half months, before I was pregnant with Brennan. David and I had just decided it was time to announce our exciting and long-awaited news when the miscarriage occurred. Suddenly we found ourselves "unannouncing" the news to those family and close friends we had just told.

People were sad and disappointed for us. Everyone, including the clinic staff, encouraged us with words such as, "You can have another baby." But that didn't help me very much; if anything, it added to the hurt. I needed first to have an acknowledgment of my pain and loss. However, David found those same words did ease some of his pain.

He or she (we never knew) was our first baby, our first pregnancy. We never felt the kicks or watched the physical changes as our baby grew, but nevertheless we felt an intense loss and an emptiness after the miscarriage.

We realized much later that we had not talked through that experience as well as we should have. It bothered David more and for a longer period of time. He had been very anxious to have a baby, but I had been unsure about the timing, so we had different reactions to the miscarriage. To keep our relationship strong, we had to talk about those differences and recognize that we grieved and reacted individually.

5

STILLBIRTH

If your baby was stillborn, it means that you had to say goodbye even before you had the chance to say hello. The immediate and intense pain of experiencing a stillbirth comes from the abrupt change of feeling euphoric and high with anticipation to the unbelievable blow of hopes dashed. All at once you have to face the reality that the baby who was kicking and obviously so alive now has died.

A stillbirth is the death of a baby anytime between twenty weeks of gestation and birth. Approximately one of every 100 babies is born dead. Most often the baby has died before the onset of labor, while the rest die during labor or at the last moment before delivery. Sometimes death is attributed to a lack of oxygen: maybe the cord was not attached correctly, was compressed or was around the baby's neck. Other times there was a problem with the placenta: it might have separated from the uterus or did not provide enough nourishment. Or death could have been due to complications from physical or genetic abnormalities. The reason for the death is unknown in other cases.

Talk with your medical attendant about what might have gone wrong in your situation. If you are concerned about the possibility of reoccurrence or genetic problems—which can be determined through genetic testing—you can consult with your doctor or a genetic counselor regarding future pregnancies.

We were told that our baby has died, but the pregnancy has to continue. How can we possibly handle this?

When parents learn their baby has died before the delivery, often they are told that for medical reasons the mother must carry the baby until either she goes into labor naturally or is closer to the due date. If this is the case for you, most likely it will be difficult and hard to understand why you have to do this. You will have to deal not only with your disbelief and grief, but you also will have to handle people's well intentioned questions and comments about your baby and the due date. You both might feel like hibernating until it is all over. It could be very beneficial at this time if you seek support and comfort from people close to you and/or professionals.

There are some things you can do to begin working through

this. Acknowledge how important this baby is to you: in spite of the fact that you know s/he is dead, do not minimize that importance. Probably you already feel attached and have love for your baby, so it does not help to think, "If I don't see or name my baby I won't get so attached, and I'll be able to forget sooner." Think carefully about whether you want to deny yourselves this chance to be physically and emotionally close with your baby.

David and I did not have much time to prepare ourselves for Brennan's death. However, during those four hours between the time we received the news that he was dead and when I delivered, we did cry, share our sorrow and talk about what we would name him, what to do about baptism, who we needed for support and whether I would stay on the maternity floor after delivery. We didn't allow ourselves to deny his importance to us at the time, and we're thankful for that.

NEONATAL DEATH

If your baby died after being born alive, you probably felt intensely sad, angry and bewildered. The anxious time waiting while your child struggled to live no doubt seemed like an eternity. You experienced the joy of giving birth, only to hear so abruptly that something was wrong.

Neonatal death is defined as the death of a baby anytime between birth and four weeks. National Center for Health statistics from 1978 put the number of U.S. neonatal deaths at 31,618 (9.5 deaths per 1000 live births).

Prematurity is a common cause of neonatal death, because the child is born with underdeveloped organs or a variety of other complications. Abnormality and birth defects might minimize the baby's chances for survival. An infant can look normal but have a congenital heart problem, a brain disorder or other internal problems. Or a baby might have malformed features or genetic problems.

When the baby is born with problems, emergency measures are taken that often include whisking the baby away to a neonatal intensive care unit or maybe another hospital. Many parents are separated from their baby, sometimes even before they have a chance to see or hold him or her.

Maybe your baby died shortly after birth, or you might have

waited helplessly for hours, days or weeks while s/he was treated. If you did not see or hold your baby before s/he died, you might feel even more agony because you can only imagine what your child looked like.

If you were told that your baby had some physical problems or deformities, you might have been afraid to look at him or her. Looking at your child, even if s/he has already died, you probably will see good features to remember, feel that the deformity is not as difficult to look at as you had feared and thus find some comfort. Frequently, parents who imagined that their baby looked terrible and were afraid to see him or her had a sense of relief when they did see their child.

Both now and later you will need the support of your partner and other loved ones, especially as you grope to accept what has happened and to begin to recover from it.

I feel guilty that I (we) gave birth to a child who was born prematurely, was deformed or couldn't survive.

It is common for parents to have some guilt feelings and a sense of failure when they have not delivered a healthy, normal infant. It is understandable, but it does not make it any easier to accept. Sometimes things happen that are out of one's control. Your energy should be spent on coping, grieving and working toward acceptance and recovery rather than feeling guilty. This will not be easy to do and will take considerable time and effort.

DECISIONS
YOU MIGHT FACE
RIGHT AWAY

You face many decisions after your baby has died. Depending upon the circumstances and your personal preferences, a number of options are available to you during the next few trying hours and days. Most of the major decisions you will have to deal with are presented in the following pages. Remember, there are no "correct" decisions; whatever you decide is right for you.

How can I possibly make all of these decisions?

Try to make them slowly and one at a time. They do not all have to be decided immediately. For example, a decision about a memorial service can be put off for a day or so. It also is helpful to make your decisions together.

Consider asking some close relatives, clergy or friends to assist you and support you at this time. You do not have to be all alone in your anguish as you struggle to come to decisions and make choices. Call someone right away to join you, if you feel the need.

The two of you will need private time together, a chance to talk things through. If you want more time alone, tell those around you. Do not worry about offending the hospital staff or friends and relatives, because they want to do what is best for you and will understand your needs if you tell them. If you want to be together through the night, tell the staff about that, too.

Our family and friends were a tremendous help and

comfort right from the beginning. We needed their support and are very thankful that we could ask for it and that they gave it willingly. We also spent much time alone with each other; we needed that, too.

Here are some concerns that you might have which need decisions:

Seeing and holding your baby

Seeing and holding your baby can be a most special time which can provide you with memories for the lonely days and years ahead, give you a chance to share your love for your little one and help you begin to accept the reality of your baby's death. Do not make a hasty decision; talk this over at length. If at first you choose not to see your child, then later change your mind, tell the staff; it usually is not too late even if it is a day or two later. You might find it difficult to mourn and accept your baby's death if you have never seen him or her.

You might be afraid to see your dead or dying baby because you imagine how terrible s/he will look. But you probably will find that as this baby's parent, you will have feelings of love, no matter what the appearance. Ask the hospital staff to prepare you for how your baby will look.

If you do hold your baby, ask to have some time alone with him or her. Unwrap the baby, so you will have a full memory; check fingers and toes, to remember the distinct features that make him or her unique and yours. Hold your baby for as long as you want; the experience of being close to your child is limited to a short time. If you feel the desire or need to hold or see your baby a day or two after the delivery, tell the hospital staff.

You might think about asking your other children, special family or friends if they want to see or hold your baby, because they have shared your joy and they too had dreams for this child. They also are left with a void now. This involvement is good for them and will help all of you to accept the loss of this real child and support one another now and in the future.

Maybe you chose not to see or hold your baby or did not get the chance to do so. If now you have a strong desire to know what your baby looked like and pictures are not available, you might consider asking your medical attendant or nurses to describe him or her. Maybe you feel o.k. that you did not see or hold your baby. Or you might regret it. Whatever you feel, try not to guilt yourself or others for a decision that has been made and cannot be undone.

David and I treasured the opportunity to hold Brennan in our arms as we lovingly said hello and began to say good-bye. I remember seeing and holding him as a most joyous moment in my life, even amidst all the pain. I always will be thankful that at least I had that. I know of parents who didn't get this chance and sadly regret it.

The baby David and I lost because of the miscarriage was not formed well enough to recognize as a baby. We did see the tissue, and although it was not pleasant, it helped us to accept the reality that the pregnancy was over and the baby had died.

Taking a picture

Choosing to have a picture taken, unless you had an early miscarriage, can provide you with a concrete memento of your baby. Even if you think you do not want a picture now, someday you might wish you had one and then it will be too late. The hospital staff probably is equipped to take a picture; you can ask the staff to do that for you and to keep it on file, in case you want it later but not now.

If your baby has some deformities, you might feel uneasy about having a picture taken. Something for you to remember when deciding is that s/he is your baby and it is all right to want to preserve the memory with a picture.

David and I felt uncomfortable when we were asked if we wanted a picture taken. In my heart I knew I wanted one, but I couldn't agree to it at the time. Now, I wish I had a photo, any photo, but especially one of us holding Brennan. I have only my memory, which is fading over time, and I have nothing tangible. I also feel badly that my family and friends didn't see Brennan and can't even see him in a picture.

Naming your baby

By giving your baby a name, you officially acknowledge the birth and his or her place in your family. You might find this decision more difficult if you had a miscarriage or a premature baby, but it still can be appropriate because it says to you and to the world that this was your baby.

When naming your baby, think about using the name you had chosen (if you did have one ready), because that name really belongs to this baby. Another name—for a future child—will be special for that baby. One child can never replace another and naming the baby might help to avoid that temptation. If you did not know the baby's sex, a name that can be either male or female, such as Pat, Erin or Chris, can be used.

You might fear that if you give your baby a name you will feel too much pain and will become too attached. But if you loved, wanted and carried your baby for any length of time, you probably have become attached; be careful not to deny this. You cannot really minimize the pain and have a healthy recovery by denying the baby's importance. Giving him or her a name recognizes that importance. If you do not name your baby right away, you still can do so in a week, a month or anytime that is good for you. You do not need to rush into that decision if you are unsure.

> *David and I are glad we named Brennan. When we use the name Brennan, it helps us and others to talk about the baby, the pregnancy, the delivery and our feelings. We realize his importance in our lives and that he was probably our first son.*
>
> *We did not name our baby who died because of miscarriage, and to a degree we did deny that baby's importance. Since it was such an early miscarriage, we didn't even consider naming the baby. I feel certain that if our baby had been more developed at the time of death, or if it were to happen to us today, we would have named him or her.*

Baptism

What you ultimately decide about baptism depends on your religious beliefs and your personal needs. Many denominations do not baptize any child, others do not baptize a baby who has died.

Baptism might be a personal comfort for you even if you have always thought of it as only for the living. You might find a prayer or a blessing for your baby to be meaningful and comforting. Consider talking with the hospital chaplain or your clergy before you make this decision.

David and I made the personal choice not to baptize Brennan, because we feel baptism is for the living and we believe that God will bless and care for him even without baptism.

Notifying family and friends

It will not be easy for you to call people and tell them your baby has died, since they have been waiting to hear good news. Feel free to call a few people and ask them to tell others; it is a way they can help and it can minimize some of the pain for you. You most likely will feel a little better once everyone has been told.

Sending an announcement of your baby's birth and death is one way to notify out-of-town friends and relatives. This can be done in a simple and sensitive manner and can relieve you from the pressure of telling everyone individually.

An example of this type of announcement is: "We are sad to tell you that our son, Brennan William Ilse, was born and died on November 2, 1981. This baby meant so much to us. We hope you will understand and share in our sorrow and loss."

People will be quite stunned with this news and will have different reactions, anything from an outburst of emotion, to tears, to total silence or a combination of these. They might say hasty words that you will not find appropriate or helpful. Try not to take these reactions personally and be aware that many people have a hard time dealing with death and do not know what to say or how to help.

David and I called many people during that first day, and even though it was extremely painful, I found it did get a little easier to talk about after awhile. David called one of his brothers who then called some of the other family members, and a neighbor called the rest of our neighborhood. Even though we didn't have to tell everyone ourselves, we were thoroughly drained after repeating the story a few times. I'm glad I made some of those calls, because it helped to prepare me for re-entering the world and the fact that I would have to talk about Brennan's death. This also helped me to continue to accept the fact that he really had died.

We felt we needed to notify our family and close friends within the first week or so, because we thought that would aid us in accepting the reality and finality and give us the ability to move on.

Mother staying on the maternity floor or moving to another area

As a patient in the hospital recovering from the birth, mom, you have the right to choose where you will stay after delivery. Most hospitals will offer a choice of where you will room, but if it is not brought up, tell the staff what you prefer.

You might find it hard to be on the maternity floor, because seeing the babies and hearing the crying is painful. Or you might need to be there because you feel it will help you accept and not "run away" from other babies; this could be hopeful amidst your grief. The experienced care from the obstetrics staff also can be helpful for you at this time.

I chose to move to another floor after I delivered Brennan, because I was afraid to hear babies crying and I didn't want to see the happy new mothers. I needed quiet time with David, away from that environment.

I was not hospitalized when I had my miscarriage. I was treated in the emergency room and released within a half hour.

14

Dad staying with mom while in the hospital

You have the right to be together at this time. If a private room is available, dad might consider staying overnight. Most hospitals will allow this, but if the staff does not offer, you can ask. This can be an especially close time for you, a time to grieve and comfort each other.

Perhaps you could not stay together because your baby was born alive, then transferred to another hospital and dad was encouraged to be with the baby. This probably was a very anxious time, with parents separated, worrying about the baby and both probably feeling helpless.

> *That first night was extraordinarily difficult for us. We did stay together and were able to share our pain. We felt it was so necessary that we were together in our shock and disbelief.*
>
> *We also used the time in the hospital to ask questions, review the birth with our medical attendant and talk about anxieties for the next time and our future plans.*

Autopsy

You might consider an autopsy, if you feel a need to know what went wrong and whether the baby was healthy. This, of course, depends on your religious and personal beliefs. A full autopsy report is not available for a number of weeks; preliminary results, however, might only take a week or two. Go over the autopsy report thoroughly with your medical attendant to get your questions answered and know that quite often what went wrong cannot be determined.

> *David and I learned that Brennan was healthy. According to our medical attendant, the problem probably was due to the umbilical cord not being attached in the best place, so the major arteries were easily exposed to pressure; during the last hours the arteries had been compressed*

15

and the blood and oxygen supply was cut off. We were re-lieved to know that he was healthy, and there was some comfort in knowing that the problem was rare and not likely to occur again.

Cremation or burial

Decide what fits your preference and budget when you make this personal decision. Whether you choose cremation or burial, try to be aware of possible future needs, such as wanting a memorial site to visit. Or maybe what is best for you is a special place to scatter the ashes of cremation.

Either a full funeral or cremation for babies can be arranged through most funeral homes. The price range varies from approximately $75 to $2,000, depending upon the service provided and the area where you live. It is a good idea for you, or someone else, to call funeral directors to discuss options, prices and to get suggestions. The funeral director understands what you are going through and can assist you in your planning.

David and I chose to cremate Brennan, because we plan cremation for ourselves. We scattered Brennan's ashes in a river, along with some flowers, as we said our good-byes. It was a place that was beautiful and special to us. We have a different feeling for that place now when we visit it; there still are some good feelings, but we also have very intense and sad moments.

Funeral-memorial service

Funeral-memorial services are for the living—for you, your family and close friends to acknowledge that this person was born into your family. It also is helpful for your family to be able to share in your sorrow, sadness and grief, along with saying goodbye to their loved one. They can be of support to you, whether you choose burial or cremation. Consider having a ceremony or a service that includes close family and friends.

If your decision is for a service, it is good for both parents to plan it and for both to be there. Wait until mom is out of the hospital (unless you choose to have the service in the hospital chapel). You will find it helpful to take time to think this decision through and choose what both of you really want, then make the proper arrangements.

After the service, it can be comforting to share a meal or some time together with people close to you, because this might be a difficult time to be alone.

> *We invited family and a few friends to join us in an informal service as we said goodbye to Brennan and scattered his ashes. It was very comforting for us to have these special people with us. Their support meant a lot to us. Afterwards we all went to a relative's house for dinner and a chance to talk. We were especially reminded at that time how fortunate we were to have such loving family and friends.*

Length of hospital stay

You will need to think about where you will recover fastest. Talk with your medical attendant to decide when it is best for you to go home. The amount of time you spend in the hospital will depend on your health and the type of delivery. You might feel you will recover faster at home, or you might need or want the hospital care.

> *I found a short stay in the hospital was what I needed. I left within 24 hours of the delivery, because I felt o.k. physically and I wanted to be at home.*

Leaving the hospital

One of the hardest things you both will have to do is leave the hospital without your baby. Your empty arms will just ache. You also might be afraid to face that special, now empty, room at home.

Mom, you might want to carry something when you leave to go home. A keepsake—such as the blanket the baby was wrapped in, the armband, a birth certificate, a footprint, a lock of hair, a record of weight and length—might be comforting for you to carry. Or dad, you can bring flowers or a plant for mom to hold. Some parents, on

17

the other hand, might feel too much pain to carry a keepsake. You might need to have empty arms since empty is how you feel.

David brought me yellow roses when I left the hospital. Even though that was far from what I had planned, at least it was comforting and I did appreciate his thoughtfulness.

THE
FIRST DAYS
AND WEEKS

Initial reactions

The minutes, hours and days have a tendency to jumble together, and you are probably feeling disoriented, confused and very vulnerable. By now your shock is probably beginning to wear off and the pain, loneliness and other intense emotions will follow. You might feel extremely sad one moment and full of anger at the "unfairness of it all" the next; this is common.

You might find yourself sighing or moaning often. Many people describe a heaviness and tightness in the chest; it might feel like a real heartache to you. These are normal grief reactions when an intense emotional trauma hits.

Many times during those first few days and weeks I remember wondering what was happening to me. I sat around and sighed continuously, experiencing such a tightness in my chest and heaviness in my heart that it was difficult to breathe at times. I didn't have any control of my emotions and had a hard time concentrating on anything— anything, that is, except my baby and our family which was robbed of an important member. Nothing else seemed to matter, not work, not other people. I couldn't make myself care about anything else. I felt as if I was not in control of my mind or my body; everything seemed to be just happening to me. I forgot many things, probably due to the fact that I just really couldn't care about anything else.

Both David and I were very confused and had a hard time making any decisions. We had a tendency to just say no to everything rather than try to make a rational decision or think the situation through. I remember that my parents called to ask if they could come to stay with us during those first few days. We said, "No, you don't have to do that. We can manage." We couldn't even think about what their suggestion meant; it was just easier to say no. After we talked it through, we wished we had said yes, because we knew it probably would help if they were there. Luckily, they did not really believe we had meant no and called back to ask us again. That time we agreed, and we were so glad they did come to be with us for a few days.

It is very easy to feel absolutely alone and helpless at this time, even if there are many people around. I have included some questions and comments to help prepare you for some of the feelings you might have and things you can do to get through these difficult days.

I feel so sad and lonely and cheated and angry. Am I going crazy?

Sometimes it can certainly feel like it. The grief you are experiencing after the death of your baby might seem endless. You might feel you are "losing it" and literally "going crazy;" this is normal and quite common. At any point in time you might feel very depressed, angry, sad, withdrawn or just drained and empty. It is not easy to accept your baby's death or to be hopeful. Eventually that will come. But probably not right away.

It is important that you express your feelings and allow yourself to grieve in whatever way you need to. You probably will feel healthier if you express your emotions and do not keep them inside; everyone copes differently. You might be tired and lethargic, might need to get busy right away or might need to scream the pain and anguish out loud. Do not box yourself in, as if you have to fit a pattern.

The stages of grief that you will probably experience are *shock, denial, bargaining, anger, sadness, disorganization, guilt, loneliness, acceptance* and *recovery.* It is common to bounce around and experience many of these emotions in one day or at any period of time. Some days will be much worse for you than others, but as time goes on those bad days will not overwhelm you as often. For now though, you can expect to feel very confused emotionally. It does not mean you are "crazy." However, if you do feel it is more than you can handle, seek assistance from someone: a family member, your clergy, a social service agency or the hospital staff.

Why me? Why us? It isn't fair!

There is not any reason why you or why us. Your loss is terrible, and you are right, it is not fair. This might be the first time a baby of yours has died, or it might not be. Each time is catastrophic, and each time the unfairness of it all strikes again.

You might wonder how this can be happening to you. It is not because you deserve it or because you are an unfit parent. It just happened. As difficult as that is for you to accept, it is true.

You might have a hard time coming to terms with this tragedy in relationship to your religious faith. You might feel angry with God, as many people do when confronted with tragedy. You will need to resolve your feelings and any anger, blame or betrayal you are experiencing. Take the time to talk this out, with your clergy, family or friends. Support can come for you now from your religious community and your faith.

Other people's comments might help or confuse you. Typical ones are, "God must have thought she was pretty special to have wanted her with Him," "God did not 'take' her, He was there to 'receive' her," "God is hurting as much as you are. He is not responsible for her death," and "He needed some young angels, too."

You soon will be aware of the conflicting beliefs people have concerning God's role in your baby's death. Once you have a sense of your own personal philosophy, comments from others will not trouble you.

How will we react toward each other? My partner does not seem to understand how I'm feeling.

Everyone grieves differently, because everyone has individual needs. Each parent experiences the loss in a unique and personal way.

Mother

Mom, you probably have had a chance to experience and feel your baby move and grow. The bond you had most likely was very strong. You not only lost a baby, but you might feel as if you lost part of yourself. You also might feel you "failed," failed in the sense of not producing a child who could live and as a couple not succeeding at something that apparently everyone else can do successfully.

The emptiness you feel inside after your baby leaves your body is something that only mothers can relate to. You ache for your baby, and your body acts as if the baby still is alive (probably your breasts are prepared to nurse and the hormone secretion increases your emotional intensity). Your maternal love for your baby most likely began long before s/he was ever born (or died). Your hopes, dreams and fantasies for this person were very real. You have not only lost a baby, but a future with this special and unique son or daughter.

You might feel very alone with your grief sometimes. People do not always know what to say or how to help. Your partner might not understand the full impact this tragedy has on you. You will need to talk about this, probably for a long time. There hardly will be a day, especially in the beginning, when you do not think about your baby. Be gentle with yourself.

You most likely will stay at home for awhile to recover. If you do go back to work soon, or on to other activities and interests, it will be awkward to talk with people. They will want to know how you are doing but might be afraid to even bring up the subject. You, yourself, also might have a problem bringing up the subject; that is natural. But if it is important for you to talk to someone about this and they do not bring it up, you might have to force yourself to do it.

Father

Dad, most likely you want to take care of your partner, to offer support and love to help her heal and to shelter her from pain. At the same time you will have your own sadness and grief. Try to allow yourself to express feelings and to get support from others. You have a difficult role to handle, and this will be a very emotionally trying time for you, too.

You probably will feel drained and confused, as does your partner. You were probably looking forward to getting to know your baby; the kicks and heartbeat had been exciting signs of good things to come. You could only experience the loss through her and for yourself, so it is doubly hard. You might want to be "strong," yet you might feel like crying. Possibly she will want to talk about the baby, the delivery and the death more than you will. As agonizing as it might be to discuss, you will feel better talking it through. Crying in front of her and showing other emotions can help you, and your partner will know that you are hurting, too, so she will not feel so alone.

In the beginning it will not be easy for you, dad, as you go back to work and face people so soon. They will want to know more about your baby's death and what happened but might be afraid to ask. You probably will have to bring up the subject many times in those first few days. Also, people tend to ask how mom is and might not inquire how you are doing and feeling. Do not pretend you are o.k. if you are not; allow yourself to tell people how you really are doing. Be aware that you are grieving, too; you have every reason to be sad, angry, disoriented or even disinterested in your work at this time.

Both Parents

Both of you should try not to feel frustrated if you seem to be on different timetables and have different needs. This is not unusual and, in fact, can work for your benefit. Sometimes one might feel unusually good, while the other one is really depressed. Do not expect too much from each other during this time. As long as you talk and keep your lines of communication open, you can work this out together. The key is to be honest and direct with each other and to look to others for support when you need it. It is easy to jump to conclusions and make assumptions that can cause problems in your relationship. You might have thoughts such as "I better not tell him how sad I am today," or "She looks like she is in a good mood and would rather not hear any more about it now."

When feelings are not shared, you might feel very lonely. Be sure to let your partner know what you want. Somedays you will want to talk, or to have a shoulder to cry on; other days you will not want to talk about it, but to think about something else. Communicate this to each other, and it is very likely that your relationship will grow and strengthen. The loss of your baby is very stressful, and you will need a strong partnership to recover and stay healthy. Many couples find this time quite trying on their relationship. Give yourself permission to seek professional help if there is undue tension and if you feel you cannot handle it alone.

I remember sitting at home many days, alone, feeling sad and sorry for myself. I tried to protect David by not discussing the topic that was so heavy on my mind. What began to happen was that the burden kept getting heavier, and I felt like it was all on me. When I finally would break down and tell David what I had been thinking, or how I had been missing Brennan, he admitted he had been feeling the same way. We would talk about it for awhile, and that always seemed to ease my burden.

Am I a parent or not?

If this was your first child, you might be unsure. You probably realize that you are not the same as before you became pregnant, but still you are not the "practicing" parents you had expected to be. You have spent months getting ready to be the parents of this baby. Now here you are, a mom or dad, with no baby.

You will want people to acknowledge that your baby died, so you could have urges to shout from the rooftops or wear a sign saying "I am a parent," or "My baby died." You are different because of this, and you never again will be quite the same.

It might be helpful for others and for you to accept your parenthood and talk about your baby. Others will pick up on the cue that you want to talk about it and not ignore it (if indeed that is what you want). You will find other mothers who will talk about delivery, sickness during pregnancy and other details. Fathers can talk to one another about their role, fears, support and the like.

In my opinion, I am a mother; I just don't have a baby at this time. But I have given birth, and the memory of my son lives with me, today and always. I expect people to treat David and me differently now. The problem is that I am not sure how I want that to be. People struggle with the dilemma of treating us the same as before, or as newly bereaved parents. It is painful and uncomfortable for us, just as it is for them.

It was not easy to do, but I personally found I was able to experience some of the joys of parenthood through my friends with children. I forced myself to see babies and to hold them. That helped me to get over some of the initial jealousy and anger I felt when I saw babies and pregnant mothers. I must admit, however, I still feel resentment, anger, jealousy and envy at times. The feelings are very unpredictable, and when they happen, I just allow them to. At times we have coped by avoiding families with children.

I feel so guilty. Is this normal?

Guilt probably is one of the most common and intense feelings parents have after the death of their child; it is a normal part of grief. Mom, you might spend hours going over your actions in the days before the baby died. Both of you might wonder if sexual activity was the cause. Or if you had feelings of uncertainty about whether you really wanted a child or whether the time was right, you might feel strongly responsible for your baby's death. Chances are that both of you feel guilty and you need to discuss that and learn not to blame yourselves. It is not your fault, and it is out of your control now.

I did have some guilt feelings and thought a lot about what I had done those last few days before Brennan died. I also remember feeling guilty and wondering if maybe my jogging and exercise classes had been the cause of the miscarriage. It helped to talk out these feelings with my medical attendant and with David. I came to understand that I really didn't do anything to cause either death, they just happened, and my feelings of guilt didn't help at all.

I blame my partner because our baby died.

It is not uncommon to feel your partner is to blame; blaming is a reaction to your own feelings of helplessness. Your baby's death is not your partner's fault, and your partner's thoughts and actions were not the cause.

Your anger needs to be expressed in some way, and often it is easier to lash out at your partner or someone close to you. This anger, in the form of blame, can be a very destructive force in your relationship. You both will need to be working for and with each other now. Try to have compassion for each other during this stressful time.

Again, talk these feelings through or seek help from a professional.

I feel so glad that David didn't blame me, nor did I blame him, since we already had so much to deal with. We did discuss the issue, however, and it was a relief for me to know that he didn't feel it was my fault.

I feel so vulnerable, weak and aged.

You are struck with your own mortality and humanness when someone you love dies, especially when it is your child, because parents are not supposed to outlive their children. You no doubt are feeling vulnerable and might fear you have lost some control in your life.

After Brennan died, I did not feel like being carefree and happy anymore, as I had most of my life. I felt I had experienced the kind of tragedy that was not supposed to hit until much later in my life. Yet here I was, not even 30, and my child had died. I felt tired and very aged. I did not want to be happy and jovial; I wanted to be sad and in mourning.

Sometimes the pain was so intense and overwhelming I worried it would never lessen. I found it impossible for awhile to feel strong or in control, but as time goes on, I have more days where I feel o.k., and in control. I'm at the point now where I feel good when I can get through a day without being overwhelmed by my sadness or anger. Those days are increasing.

I'm sure I still feel my baby kick. How can this be?

You are not going crazy. This is a very real phenomenon. Many mothers are quite certain that they feel the baby kick, long after the birth. As a mother whose baby has died, you might want to believe the kicks are real, because you have a need to feel life.

Often I feel what I believe is my baby kicking. At first I thought that was very strange and I worried about my sanity. After talking with other mothers, I found that this was very common, and I was relieved. I am not so afraid of these sensations now, and in fact, I try to remember the joyful times associated with those kicks.

I still look pregnant. That is too hard to handle sometimes.

You still might look pregnant even weeks after you have delivered. It is likely that people will ask you when your baby is due; your reactions will depend on the circumstances and your mood at the time. Some days you will be able to respond directly without a lot of anguish, and other days you might not even be able to answer. The emotional and hormonal transition you are experiencing will take time. Be aware that your reactions will be unpredictable and allow yourself to feel whatever emotion is within you.

Your body adjusts slowly to the fact that your pregnancy has ended. It might seem especially unfair and cruel that your body and mind take so long to accomplish this. Try to accept that the changes happen over time.

You might feel the hard part in this situation is that you have made such a sacrifice with your body and "don't have anything to show for it." You did have a baby, even if s/he did not live, and now you will have to be patient while you get back in shape. Do not rush yourself into looking and acting "unpregnant" too soon, and do not push yourself too hard to get that shape back; you will find it takes anywhere from six months to a year to recover physically. You will be happier with yourself if you work on it conscientiously and with patience.

About a month after I gave birth someone in a store asked me when my baby was due. The color rose in my cheeks and I remember stuttering, not knowing what to say. Finally, I decided to tell the truth and not make up a story as I was tempted to do. The woman seemed genuinely sad; she felt badly that she had asked. Because I was so open about it, and she had gotten over the shock, we talked about Brennan, what it was like to experience my baby's death and how I was doing. I was glad I had been able to discuss it with her. On other days, however, there was no way I could tell people the whole story, so I would say I already had my baby and walk away.

I do remember being upset that my body was such a wreck and I didn't even have a baby to make the sacrifice seem worth it. It seemed unmercifully cruel.

What do I have to live for now? Sometimes I feel like I want to die.

The question you are asking is a valid one. What *do* you have to live for? It probably feels as if your world has collapsed and not much else matters. So maybe you sometimes feel that "I should just give up."

It is very important that you find at least a reason or two to continue living. If you have a reason cemented in your mind, it will act as a buffer and will help you when urges arise to "give up."

You have much to live for, if you really think about it and look at your whole life. Sometimes, when in the depths of despair, it is not easy to remember what is good in your life. Your partner, family, friends, clergy, a social worker or some other professional therapist can help you find those reasons which make your life meaningful. To work your way out of the depression and the feelings of giving up, think about what you have to look forward to tomorrow or next week. Maybe it is another child's birthday or Confirmation, a vacation or your anniversary, or a project you need to complete. Take it a day at a time and keep reminding yourself how important you are to others and how important they are to you.

You should be aware that suicidal thoughts are relatively common at this time but suicide will not bring your baby back. You might think about using the experience of your baby's death as a way to help your life have meaning.

If you feel that "I wish I would have died instead of my child," know that many others have felt this also. These feelings usually do not last, but it is a heavy burden to carry alone. Talk it out, express your emotions and do not worry if you think you are going crazy sometimes. It helps to let out your anger and emotions when you are feeling them; when emotions are kept buried inside they build up to an intensity that sometimes can lead to extreme actions.

If you feel you have not resolved your grief, or feel exceptionally depressed or suicidal, seek help immediately. There are many people who care and can be of assistance. Call a social worker, your clergy, a therapist or your local mental health center.*

*Be aware that not every professional has expertise in every problem. If your needs are not met, and you do not feel satisfied with the help you are receiving, find another professional and know that there is someone who can provide valuable assistance for you. You might have to keep looking until you find the appropriate professional.

Often a bereaved parent support group, led by a professional is a good source of help. Other parents are there who have experienced a similar situation. They can provide you with names of professionals who helped them.

I don't remember having feelings of wanting to die. It's possible that I did, but maybe I have blocked them out of my thoughts. I knew there were many reasons why I wanted to live and that I did have some things to look forward to, even if a major piece of my life was no longer there.

How do I tell my other children? Should I protect them from the truth?

Although young children lack deep understanding about death, they are experiencing many of the same emotions you are. They need to hear the truth. Share your thoughts and tears with them. They often have similar feelings of guilt that should be talked about (maybe they expressed feelings of not wanting a baby in their house or did not look forward to sharing a room). Even though you know those feelings of guilt are unrealistic, to a child they are very real. If they do not get a chance to learn that they are not responsible for their brother or sister's death, they might carry those feelings with them as they grow up.

It often is suggested to keep the children involved in the experience of the funeral, discussing how sad you are not to bring the baby home, etc. You can help to make the experience real in their minds, encourage them to begin to accept the meaning of death and make them feel loved and included. There are many books that can teach children about death; some of them are listed in the bibliography.

How will people react toward me now?

You definitely will experience mixed reactions from others. Before your baby was ever born, you had plans and dreams for his or her future as a loved member of your family. S/he existed as a real, special and unique person, one no one really knew but you. You grieve for that baby as if s/he had lived, and you grieve for the future with him or her that will never be.

Family and friends probably will not be able to fully understand, as you do, unless they have experienced a similar death. The death of an infant is most unusual and difficult for people to deal with. They have never "met," held or played with your baby. They did not feel the baby kick, and probably did not spend as many hours as you did thinking about what the baby would look like and dreaming about this baby as a member of "our family." Therefore, they have little to relate to and mainly experience the grief through you. They hurt mostly because you hurt. Many will want to comfort you and offer their support. Help them to know what would be of benefit to you. Share this with them so they can better understand.

You might find that some well-meaning people believe that since your baby did not live—or did not live very long—your attachment is less than if you had lost a two or a 20-year-old. This probably is not true, although each loss is different and unique. When your hopes, dreams, fantasies and the very real attachment came to an end after months, and sometimes years, of anticipation, the grief can be extremely intense. As one mother put it, "On a scale of one to ten, when your child dies, it is always a ten." So no matter when your baby died —three months in utero, at birth or after birth—you have every right to feel sad, angry or lonely.

Others' reactions to your news will be varied. Sometimes even close friends and family members might avoid you or the subject of your baby's death. They probably do not realize your need to talk. Or they might say things that seem trivial or are painful to you. For example, someone might tell you, "You didn't really know her anyway," "At least you have other children," "You can always have another baby." They say these things because they do not want you to hurt any more than you already do. Most people have difficulty talking about death and knowing how to comfort the survivors, so even though their comments might not be appropriate, they do not mean to hurt you.

You most likely will need to let people know when it is o.k. to talk about what happened. You will find that quite often you will have to bring up the subject or at least open the door so others will know you want to talk. If you can cope with the reality of your baby's death, others also will become more comfortable talking about it with you.

> When people told me "Have another baby," it was important for me to say, "But I'm sad about this baby. This one was important to me and having another baby won't make me forget about this one." I did appreciate that they were trying to be gentle and supportive, but it wasn't what I needed to hear at the time.
>
> We very much wanted our family and friends to bring up the subject, to acknowledge that this tragedy was an important event in our lives. It happened, and it was very painful, but we did not want to forget. Rather, we needed to come to accept and remember. We knew the pain would not magical-

ly go away if we didn't discuss it. We needed to talk about Brennan and the experience, to work through it. We felt this would help us heal, and it has.

Some Things You Can Do That Might Help

It is likely that this is one of the most painful experiences in your life, so everything probably feels overwhelming and unreal. When you are ready, there are some things you can do that might help to minimize the pain or just aid you in getting through some of the tough days.

It probably is wise not to second-guess your decisions; you are making them as wisely as you can. The best advice we heard from anyone was, "Do what you need to do, for yourselves. Don't do things for someone else. Make decisions and act according to your beliefs and needs."

Here are some suggestions for you to consider:

—Involve your family and friends immediately to share your grief and for their support. Use their strength and let them help.

—Talk about your baby, your feelings and your grief . . . and talk about it some more, to your partner, family, friends, co-workers or other bereaved parents. This was an important event in your life; it will not go away just because you ignore or try to forget it.

—When you talk about your baby, use his or her name. This makes your baby more real and recognizes the importance of this person in your life.

—Talk about the delivery, how s/he looked, your fears, any happiness, apprehension or despair you felt. If you have pictures, show them to others (if you choose to do so).

—Acknowledge your parenthood, even if this was your first child. Remember, even though your baby has died, you are a parent. Life will never be quite the same as before.

—Share the first days at home together with your partner. If dad can take some time off from work, make a point to do it so you will have those hours with each other.

—Encourage visitors soon. This might help lessen some of the emptiness you probably feel and can keep you involved in the world.

—When others ask "Is there anything we can do?" give them specific suggestions. Tell them what you need: food, company, child-care . . . or give them this book to read. They want to do something, so help them to know what you need.

—Avoid making hasty decisions about the baby's belongings and room. Do not let others take over or make decisions for you. This is part of the process of acceptance for you. You should choose whether you will put things away or leave them out. Whatever you decide, use this time (as difficult and painful as it will be) to share tears, unmet dreams and fantasies, stories of the pregnancy, etc.

—Write your feelings down, keep a journal or a memory book. Make a baby book with mementos, cards, keepsakes, etc. You can keep the memory of your baby alive with such things as a framed poem that was special to you, a set of footprints, baby pictures, a plant that was received while you were in the hospital.

—Talk to your clergy to help you understand and restore your faith in God, if you find it failing.

—Be active: exercise, walk, do something physical. It helps to release some of the anger and frustration and also is good for recovering.

—Set time aside periodically (daily, and then weekly, as time progresses) to talk with your partner. Time will pass, but still you will feel a need to talk about your baby and your grief.

—Try not to make major changes in your life before you are ready (job changes, moving or a permanent decision regarding more children). This time already is stressful. Keep as much of the rest of your life intact as you can.

—Read books (see bibliography), articles, poems, when you are ready, to help you understand, to seek comfort so you will not feel so alone.

—Call local hospitals or your local Compassionate Friends Chapter to find a grief support group that specifically helps parents whose infant has died. This will give you an opportunity to talk with other couples who have "been there;" others can offer you support, help and hope.

—Admit to yourself and to family and friends when you need help. It is not easy to ask for help or even to admit that you need it. This takes courage, but it certainly can diminish your pain and loneliness.

AFTER
SOME TIME
HAS PASSED

Some days you will feel as if you are well on the road to recovery, and on others you will feel as if you are right back in the middle of all that grief. One mother commented that she felt she would "Move one step ahead, then two steps backward." You will find this to be a very up and down emotional period. Know that you probably will feel differently from one day to the next. It does get better, the pain does lessen, although it might never go away completely.

As you come to accept your baby's death, recognize that you are beginning to recover. That is not to say you will not be angry or frustrated at times. You will continue to miss your baby and feel cheated that you are not spending your time parenting this child instead of trying to keep busy and to recover.

Hardly a day goes by when I do not think about Brennan or this tragic experience. At least now, however, I do not fall to pieces every time I think about it. I have talked about it so much that my emotions usually do not jump out and take over every time. But sometimes they do, and I cannot stop that. The memory never really fades too much, but I never want to forget, just to accept.

Here are more suggestions for concerns you probably have at this time:

What else can I do to get over this and move on in a healthy manner?

—Treat yourself to something special: a dinner out, a new outfit, a trip or a vacation.
—Know, mom, that is is likely that you will have to remain at home for awhile to recover physically from the birth. Emotionally you probably will feel better sooner if you make a point of getting involved with work, a hobby or community activities. Do not become so busy, however, that you avoid thinking about your loss and grief totally.
—Continue to exercise and work off your frustrations, along with getting yourself back in shape. It is good for your physical and mental health.
—Plan some fun activities, too, even if it seems impossible. You need to realize that life must go on. The time will come when you are ready to bring some happiness and humor back into your life, and you will feel better once that begins to happen.
—Be aware that holidays, birthdays and your due date can be very sad, lonely and trying times. Some periods that can be especially difficult are one month, six months and one year after the baby died. Many situations can trigger memories, such as seeing other babies and pregnant women.
—Tell yourself often that time will help, the pain will lessen and tomorrow will come, even if you initially do not believe it. Have hope for the future. Time and love do help to heal those deep wounds.

I am fearful of having sexual intercourse with my partner. Somehow it doesn't seem right.

Sexuality is an issue that is rarely discussed after a healthy baby is born and even less so when a baby dies. But it should be talked about.

It might seem healthy and normal for you to have sexual intercourse and be intimately close at this time. Or one or both of you might have a difficult time feeling comfortable about love making after the death of your baby. In your mind, you might link the act of intercourse with the conception of your baby who died. You might feel guilty or angry that intercourse was "the beginning or cause of this tragedy and all my pain." That could be dangerous to your relationship. Maybe it will not be easy for you to enjoy sex or intimacy if you feel you should be in mourning and not thinking about yourself. Try not to feel guilty or to think about the baby at this time; it helps if you can keep thoughts of the baby out of the bedroom. Life must go on for both of you, and you need to re-establish your relationship and restore your energy. Being close, especially now, could aid you in recovery. You deserve and need some private and warm time together. It also is important to discuss how each of you feels, and if one of you does not feel comfortable, do take things slowly. Keep the lines of communication open and be patient.

Do seek professional help if you feel unsuccessful after trying your best to work this out.

I didn't have fearful feelings about sexual intercourse. In fact, I looked forward to the intimacy of it, because it was one of the few times when thoughts of Brennan didn't overpower all my other thoughts. The closeness was comforting to me.

My friends, family and co-workers seem to have forgotten that I had this baby. No one ever asks about the baby.

After awhile— sometimes no longer than a month—people will stop bringing up the subject of your baby's death. They might feel you should be "over it" by now or just want to protect you from those painful memories. They might believe that by bringing it up they will hurt you. If you need to talk about it, you most likely will have to bring it up yourself. Let people know that you are not trying to forget your baby but to remember in as painless a way as possible.

I felt badly when people stopped asking me about Brennan, the loss and how I was doing. After not talking about it much, sometimes I wondered if I ever really was pregnant and had a baby. My body had recovered and did not look pregnant. I have little around the house to remind me of Brennan. On those days when I questioned if I had a baby, I needed to feel that pain, remember my loss and talk about it. The pain and the memories were like jolts, reminding me that, yes, it was true: I am a mother, I've had a child.

35

What about getting pregnant again? I'm afraid I will be terribly anxious and worried throughout the pregnancy.

If, for medical reasons or personal choice, you will not have another pregnancy, you might need to work with each other, your family and possibly your clergy or a professional therapist. Even more grief is involved here, the grief of all the children you will not have. You will have some heavy decisions to make and coming to terms with this major change in your life will not be easy.

If you do plan another pregnancy, you probably will wonder when it is advisable to do so. Each person is different, and your medical attendant will have a suggestion specifically for you; it will depend on your physical and emotional recovery. Just be careful that you are not trying to have another baby to take the place of the one who just died. That would not be fair to the next child or to you, because each is a unique pregnancy and a unique child with a special name and individual characteristics.

You might be nervous and not feel ready to try again for a long while. You could experience difficulty in becoming pregnant; it often takes time and patience. Consult with your medical attendant if you think it is taking too much time or if you feel that something is wrong.

Once you are pregnant again, you probably will feel anxious and excited at the same time. Chances are you will experience a good deal of fear. This pregnancy might not be an easy one, since you will think about the previous pregnancy as this baby grows. Many parents seek counseling or support during this period. You might find it especially useful to talk with other parents who have lost a baby and then given birth to another. Talk about your fears and concerns but do not forget to enjoy and allow yourself to have pleasant thoughts throughout this pregnancy. It is o.k. to be happy about this baby, even if you still feel sad about the one who died.

If you adopt or give birth, when your child arrives, you both will most likely feel a great sense of joy and pain and sadness at the same time. It will be a powerful and an emotionally-charged time. You probably will miss your other baby; it is good to acknowledge this and to enjoy your new baby. You waited a long time for this special gift and deserve some happiness.

RECOVERING

Even though you want to hear, and believe, that you will recover quickly and completely from the death of your child, that might not be the case. It is a very painful process that takes time and much work. Recovery has a different meaning for everyone. For you, it might mean less frequent crying, making it through many days feeling somewhat normal or remembering your baby without so much pain. Maybe you will return to work or other activities as you reconstruct your life, allowing other things to become important to you again.

Some of the pain might always be with you, as will the memory of your baby. It probably will be healthy for you to come to accept the death, to continue to express your sadness, anger and other feelings and to fondly, warmly and lovingly remember your baby.

There is no magic date, such as a one or ten year anniversary, when you will feel instantly healed and recovered. Just because one year has passed, do not expect that the bad days are all over for you. Most of the hurt probably has lessened, but there still will be days when you are overcome by sadness and pain. Allow that to happen.

Other people often give the message: "Now that it has been a year, you should be over it." Sometimes they say that after only a few months. Let them know you still have bad times, but yes, you also have good times. People who have experienced a death themselves often understand this.

Two women I know, one 85 and the other 97, each gave birth to a number of children. Both had several children who lived, and both had a baby who had died. They still think of their baby who didn't live, and their eyes well up with tears when they talk about their son or daughter and what that person might have been like today.

I do believe that now, eight months later, I am well on my way to feeling recovered. There are many people and activities that once again are important to me. I feel that Brennan's death is in proper perspective with the rest of my life. When I remember him I still am deeply saddened, will never forget and I know the pain never will go away completely. But I do have happiness in my life, and I have many good days.

I found some comfort in the following poem written by Abraham Lincoln, a very fine and sensitive man who had three sons who died: Edward, age 4; William, 11; and Thomas, age 18.

"In this sad world of ours, sorrow comes to all . . .
It comes with bitterest agony . . .
Perfect relief is not possible, except with time.

You cannot now realize that you will even feel better . . .
And yet this is a mistake.
You are sure to be happy again.

To know this, which is certainly true,
Will make you become less miserable now.
I have experienced enough to know what I say."

Abraham Lincoln

Hope . . . Time . . . Love . . . Healing

Tomorrow will come. The pain will ease. But you will never forget your precious child. It takes hope and time and love for the healing to take place. Remember along the way to accept, but not forget.

WHAT FAMILY
AND FRIENDS
CAN DO

Loved ones, this is for you. It is not easy to know what to do or say to someone who has lost his or her baby. Death reminds us all of our own humanness and mortality. Most of us would rather not think or talk about death. However, at this painful time in the parents' lives, they need to talk about their baby, their feelings and their concerns. When a baby dies, it seems even more difficult to deal with. All were waiting for the joyous day and now the opposite has happened.

Friends and family can aid and support the parents by encouraging them to talk. This helps them to accept the death and grieve themselves, along with sharing this intense pain with you. Ignoring the subject does *not* make it go away, nor does it make the parents feel less pain. In most cases it hurts more when people will not talk about it with the parents; this is often interpreted by parents as insensitivity or disinterest. They need to know that their loved ones are willing and interested in hearing about their experience. After all, this has been one of the most tragic and devastating events in their lives.

What can I do to help the parents?

—Offer a tear, a hug . . . a sign of love and concern.
—Listen, talk about the death and about their son or daughter. Ask questions if they want to talk. Most parents need and want to talk about their baby, their hopes and dreams with their child that has died (even if it was a miscarriage).
—Ask the parents "Do you feel like talking about it now or would later be better?"
—Realize that the parents are sad because they lost *this* baby, this

special person; he or she never can be replaced by anyone else. They had pictured their son or daughter, in their minds, learning to walk, starting school, making friends, graduating, getting married and having their own children. They did not lose "just" a baby, but a whole future.

—Comments such as "I am sorry about your baby," "I know this is a bad time for you, and I would like to help," "Please tell me what you would like me to do." "Can I bring dinner over?" and "I feel so sad" might seem trite, but they really do help.

—Comments such at "It was for the best," ". . . might have been abnormal," "You can always have another baby," "Forget it, put it behind you," tend to deny the importance of *this* baby in the parents' lives.

—Send a card, note, poem or some other personal expression of sympathy.

—Bring a plate of goodies or a casserole to the family.

—Offer to babysit, wash clothes or do some other household chores.

—Bring a book that might offer comfort or some understanding (see bibliography for suggestions).

—Give a gift certificate for a dinner or maybe a rubdown at the local spa or health club.

—Give a plant, a living bush, a tree or flowers. Sometimes living things represent continuity and a sense of future, which is so desperately needed at this time.

—Pass on names and phone numbers of others who have experienced a similar loss and seem to be coping well. There is a real need to talk with others who "have been through it."

—Ask parents about their preference regarding donating money and memorials. (I used the money friends donated to help publish this book.)

—Recognize that the parents' grief and the recovery process will be painful and will take time, lots of time. They will not be recovered or done "thinking about their baby" after a month or even a year.

—Be aware that they never again will be quite the same people you knew before they had this baby. Their lives have changed, their perspectives and goals also might be different. Recognize and respect this.

—Do discuss other topics besides their loss. Life must go on.

—Again, recognize the importance of *this* baby. The loss and pain cannot be replaced with another baby. And do make the effort to talk with them about the baby and how they are doing. Months down the road a simple "How have you been doing since your baby died?" can give much comfort.

Your assistance, comfort and support can be very influential in how the parents cope with the death of their baby and how they recover. You are important loved ones; they need you now more than ever.

NATIONAL RESOURCES

Support

AMEND
P.O. Box 2950
Hollywood, CA 90028
(313) 271-1264

Volunteer counselors offer support and encouragement to parents who have experienced neonatal death.

THE COMPASSIONATE
FRIENDS, INC.
National Headquarters
P.O. Box 1347
Oak Brook, IL 60521

A self-help organization of bereaved parents helping each other; local chapters exist.

HOPING
Sparrow Hospital
1215 East Michigan Avenue
Lansing, MI 48909

Offers support groups for parents experiencing miscarriage, stillbirth and neonatal death; parent to parent support. A borrowing library.

NATIONAL SUDDEN INFANT
DEATH SYNDROME FOUNDA-
TION
Two Metro Plaza
Suite 205
8240 Professional Place
Landover, MD 20785
(301) 459-3388

Information and referral for parents regarding crib death.

PARENTS OF PREMATURES
Houston Organization for Parent Education, Inc.
3311 Richmond, Suite 330
Houston, TX 77098
(713) 524-3089

A volunteer service organization providing support and dissemination of information regarding prematurity.

SHARE
St. John's Hospital
800 E. Carpenter Street
Springfield, IL 62702
(217) 544-6464, ext. 4500

Offers groups for parents after miscarriage, stillbirth or newborn loss. Publishes newsletter.

Childbirth

AMERICAN FOUNDATION
FOR MATERNAL AND CHILD
HEALTH, INC.
30 Beekman Place
New York, NY 10022
(212) 759-5510

ICEA (International Childbirth Education Association)
Box 20048
Minneapolis, MN 55420
(612) 854-8660

Education and support for a more satisfying birth experience. Some of the local groups sponsor services for parents after miscarriage, stillbirth and neonatal death.

NATIONAL PERINATAL
ASSOCIATION
1015 15th Street, N.W.
Suite 420
Washington, D.C. 20005
(202) 556-9222

Counseling

If you do not know how to contact a local counselor or therapist, these National Organizations might be able to give you information about someone in your area.

AMERICAN PSYCHIATRIC ASSOCIATION
1700 18th Street, N.W.
Washington, D.C. 20009
(202) 797-4900

AMERICAN PSYCHOLOGICAL ASSOCIATION
1200 17th Street, N.W.
Washington, D.C. 20036
(202) 833-7600

FAMILY SERVICE ASSOCIATION OF AMERICA
44 East 23rd Street
New York, NY 10010
(292) 674-6100

NATIONAL ASSOCIATION OF SOCIAL WORKERS
Supervisor of Registers and Directories
7981 Eastern Avenue
Silver Spring, MD 20910
(301) 565-0333

Ob-Gyn

AMERICAN ASSOCIATION OF OB-GYN
4200 E. 9th Avenue
Denver, CO 80220
(303) 394-7616

AMERICAN COLLEGE OF OB-GYN
600 Maryland Avenue, S.W.
Suite 300
Washington, D.C. 20024
(202) 638-5577

Infertility

RESOLVE, INC.
P.O. Box 474
Belmont, MA 02178
(617) 484-2424

Support and information concerning infertility.

Adoption

AASK (Aid to the Adoption of
Special Kids)
3530 Grand Avenue
Oakland, CA 94611
(415) 451-1748

ARENA (Adoption Resource
Exchange of North America)
67 Irving Place
New York, NY 10003
(212) 254-7410

CHILDREN'S BUREAU, OFFICE
OF CHILD DEVELOPMENT
Health and Human Services
P.O. Box 1182
Washington, D.C. 20013
(202) 755-7762

OURS (Organization for United
Response)
4711 30th Avenue South
Minneapolis, MN 55406

Organization of adoptive parents, providing information especially on international adoption

BIBLIOGRAPHY

After a Loss in Pregnancy, Help for Families Affected by A Miscarriage, A Stillbirth or the Loss of a Newborn, Nancy Berezin, Simon and Schuster, 1982. "Based on hundreds of interviews with women who have experienced a miscarriage, stillbirth or the loss of a newborn, the book takes an honest look at a woman's grief and at the various social forces and institutions that work for or against a recovery... provides down to earth advice for coping."

Before and After My Child Died: A Collection of Parents' Experiences, Joseph Fischhoff, M.D. and Noreen O'Brien Brohl, M.S.W., Emmons-Fairfield Publishing Co., Detroit, 1981. "A beautiful collection... that is written in human, understandable language and shows the different aspects of coping."

Bereaved Parents, Harriet Schiff, Crown Publisher, 1977. A book for parents, in any stage of grief, who have suffered the death of a child. The decisions and hardships that must be faced are presented with practical step-by-step directions on how to cope. Emphasis is on rebuilding the survivors' lives and healing.

Beyond Sorrow, Herb and Mary Montgomery, Winston Press, 1977. A short, quick reading book with a Christian perspective that uses the Scriptures to help understand some of the questions that people have after a tragedy.

But For Our Grief: A Look at How Comfort Comes, June Taylor, Holman Publishing, 1977. "A book filled with insight, a personal pilgrimage from numbing pain and doubt, through prayerful searching, to restored peace and faith. The author draws upon the personal insights with her chief reliance on the words of the Bible."

Coping With a Miscarriage, Hank Pizner & Christine O'Brien Palinski, Dial Press, 1979. A thorough book that presents a clear, reassuring explanation of the causes, medical procedures and treatments of a miscarriage, along with guidelines for selecting a doctor and treatment plan. It also addresses the emotional issues for both men and women, their reactions and suggestions for seeking support. Written in laypersons' words, very frank and easy to read.

The Courage to Grieve - Creative Living, Recovery and Growth through Grief, Judy Tatelbaum, Lippincott & Crowell, 1980. This book discusses things to be done after a death occurs.

47

Don't Take My Grief Away From Me, Doug Manning, Creative Marketing, P.O. Box 2423, Springfield, IL 62705. A practical, supportive and informative book for grieving family members.

Death: The Final Stage of Growth, Elisabeth Kubler-Ross, Prentice-Hall, 1975. A book of essays presenting death from many different points of view, it will help you examine your own views about life and death.

The Denial of Death, Ernest Becker, Free Press, 1973. This book provides the thought-provoking philosophy about death: our lifelong struggle against death is at the heart of human life and all of our activities.

For the Living, Edgar N. Jackson, Channel Press, 1963. The meaning of grief and the social ceremonies which deal with death and loss are presented.

Getting Through the Night, Eugenia Price, New York Dial Press, 1982. "This is a well-written book for those who have experienced the loss of a loved one. It's purpose is to give anyone who is in grief, for whatever reason, an assurance that there is help available—God's help."

Good Grief, Granger Westberg, Philadelphia, Fortress Press, 1962. A general book about the stages of grief whenever people lose someone or something important in their lives.

How to Survive the Loss of a Love, Melba Colgrove, Bantam, 1976. The author discusses 58 ways to help you cope with loss, including the death of a loved one.

How to Survive the Loss of a Loved One, Melba Colgrove, Bloomfield & McWilliams, Bantam, 1977. A short, readable book with poetry and practical suggestions.

In the Midst of Winter: Selections from the Literature of Mourning, Mary J. Moffat, Random, 1982. This book is an "anthology of writings about the process of mourning . . . it contains poems, diaries, letters . . . and reveals the nature and progress of grief."

Life is Goodbye, Life is Hello. Alla Bozarth Campbell, Compcare Publications, 1982. The book provides a hopeful message and is written to help people grieve "well" through all kinds of loss.

Living When a Loved One Has Died, Earl A. Grollman, Beacon Press, 1977. Dr. Grollman, regarded as one of the foremost counselors on death, dying and bereavement, also is a clergyman who writes with a simple compassion, a comfort to help people go on living wisely.

Love is Stronger than Death, Peter J. Kreeft, Harper-Row, 1979. This book addresses such questions as what is death and why do we die, in a Christian inspirational and philosophical manner.

Maternal-Infant Bonding, Marshall H. Klaus and John H. Kemnel, C.V. Mosby Co., 1976. This book is especially written for the professionals who work with bereaved parents. It gives a good background and history of maternal-infant bonding.

Motherhood and Mourning, Larry Peppers and Ronald Knapp, Praeger, 1980. A book written for mothers who have lost their babies and for those who help them cope with their grief. Information is offered, along with actual accounts of women who have gone through this experience, covering such topics as characteristics of grieving mothers, stages of maternal grief and marital conflicts following infant death.

Mourning Song, Joyce Landorf, Fleming H. Rewell Co., 1974. A moving book

48

written by a woman who lost her infant son, grandfather and mother in a year's time. The author shares her Christian beliefs, her pain and sorrow and an understanding of how to work through grief in healthy ways.

Newborn Death, Joy and Marv Johnson, Centering Corporation, 1982. This short book is written for parents experiencing stillbirth, miscarriage or newborn death.

Nothing to Cry About, Barbara J. Berg, Harper & Row, 1981. A painful story of a mother who experienced a miscarriage, a stillbirth and later infertility and the problems she faced with some insensitive medical professionals.

On Death and Dying, Elisabeth Kubler-Ross, Macmillan, 1969. The "classic Kubler-Ross" discusses the five stages of death and dying: denial and isolation, anger, bargaining, depression and acceptance.

Our Life With Caleb, Jared and Alice Massanari, Fortress Press, 1976. A mother and father tell their story of life with their son Caleb who lived for five months in an intensive care nursery. It can aid in understanding the trials of caring for a premature baby.

Premature Babies: A Handbook for Parents, Sherry Mance, Arbor House, 1982. This comprehensive guide provides personal stories, practical advice and the latest medical findings, written by parents.

Questions and Answers on Death and Dying, Elisabeth Kubler-Ross, Macmillan, 1974. The author provides discussion and answers to the most frequently asked questions about death and dying: for example, telling a person s/he is dying, how to approach a dying person, suicide, euthansia and sudden death, funerals and other necessary arrangements and the family problems before and after death has occurred.

Rachael, Arthur A. Smith, Morehouse-Barlow, 1975. A clergyman and father addresses the feelings and problems of his grief as he tells of the sudden, unexplained death of his ten-year-old daughter. He discusses anger, frustration and depression from a father's viewpoint. This is reassuring especially to the newly bereaved as they struggle with feelings of loneliness and a variety of conflicting emotions.

Recovering from the Loss of a Child, Katherine Fair Donnelly, Macmillan, 1982. This book offers many experiences and insights of parents who have experienced the loss of a child.

Surviving Pregnancy Loss, Rochelle Friedman, M.D., Bonnie Gradstein, M.D., Little, Brown & Co., 1982. The book provides a comprehensive discussion of the physical and emotional consequences of pregnancy loss, stories of women and the exploration of options for the future.

Swimmer in the Secret Sea, William Katzwinkle, Avon, 1975. A moving story of a stillbirth, this short novel tells about a young father and his unborn son.

The Ultimate Loss, Coping with the Death of a Child, Joan Bordow, Beaufort Books, Inc., 1982. This book includes many case histories and commentaries, discusses how to cope and offers the professionals' point of view.

What Helped Me When My Loved One Died, Earl A. Grollman, Beacon Press, 1981. The author presents personal stories of many who have mourned the death of a loved one due to accidental death, long illness, suicide, SIDS and war.

When Bad Things Happen to Good People, Harold S. Kushner, Schoeken Books, 1981. This book encourages reaching out to God when tragedy strikes to find comfort and hope without blaming Him. It brings faith, inspiration and promise that people are not alone with their pain and grief.

When Going to Pieces Holds You Together, William A. Miller, Augsburg, 1976. Dealing with the experience of personal loss, the philosophy points out that going to pieces at the time of loss is a normal and natural human experience, and that it might be the very thing that will hold people together as they work through the grief process.

When Pregnancy Fails: Families Coping with Miscarriage, Stillbirth and Infant Death, Susan Borg and Judith Lasker, Beacon Press, 1981. This comprehensive book presents fears, feelings, problems, suggestions and explanations for parents and includes a good resource guide and an extensive bibliography.

When Someone Dies, Edgar N. Jackson, Fortress Press, 1971. "Grief is not an enemy, but a process that leads to healthful recovery from loss. In this book, the author emphasizes the skills and insights that help people work through this process into a smooth and sustained life."

You and Your Grief, Edgar N. Jackson, Channel Press, 1962. A short, readable book that gives the grieving person hope to "emerge" from the depths of the tragedy, encourages people to take the power of life and use it to deal with death, offers suggestions to help with grieving children and encourages the bereaved to let themselves be helped and to "feel."

Helping Children Deal with Death

About Dying. An Open Book for Parents and Children Together, S.B. Stein, Walker and Co., 1974. This is one of an outstanding series of "open family books" for parents and children to read together. It offers suggestions for parents in helping children understand and cope with death. The story tells of a bird that dies, then about a grandfather who dies and concludes with a discussion of how parents can help children to cope with such events.

Beginnings, Helen Galinsky, Houghton Mifflin, 1976. A young mother's story of two sons born prematurely, one who survives and the second one who does not. It contains good descriptions of how the first son reacts to his brother's death.

Children and Dying: An Exploration and Selective Bibliographies, R. L. Carr, Health Sciences Publishing Corporation, 1974.

Helping Your Child to Understand About Death, A. W. M. Wolf, Child Study Press, 1973.

Learning to Say Goodbye, Eda LeShan, Avon, 1978.

Living with an Empty Chair—A Guide Through Grief, Roberta Times, Mandala Press, 1977.

Should the Children Know? Encounters with Death in the Lives of Children, Marguerita Rudolph, Schocken Books, 1978. The book "shows how the very young can and should be taught about death at school and at home — through books, the care of plants and animals, and direct experience with human death. It is sensitive and sensible, good for teachers and parents."

Talking About Death: A Dialogue Between Parent and Child, Earl A. Grollman, Beacon Press, 1976. Death is explained in a clear, easily understandable format. It gives examples of what fears/questions children have and how parents can respond honestly and directly; a resource bibliography is included.

Telling a Child About Death, Edgar N. Jackson, Channel Books, 1965. The author discusses "when to talk about death to children, what to say, how children of different ages will react and how to understand the nature of a child's grief."

Tell Me Papa, Joy and Marvin Johnson, Highly Specialized Publishing, 1980.

What to Tell Your Child: About Birth, Illness, Death, Divorce and Other Family Crises, Helen S. Arnstein, Condor Publishing Co., 1978.

Children's Fiction - Books Concerning Death

Annie & The Old One, Margaret Wise Brown, Boston, Little, Brown, 1971.	Elementary
Charlotte's Web, E. B. White, New York, Harper & Row, 1952.	Elementary
The Dead Bird, Margaret Wise Brown, New York, Scott, 1958.	Preschool
Death Be Not Proud, J. Gunther, New York, Harper, 1949.	Secondary
Growing Time, S. Warburg, Boston, Houghton, Mifflin, 1969.	Elementary
Sunshine, N. Klein, New York, Avon, 1974.	Secondary
The Tenth Good Thing About Barney, J. Viorst, New York, Atheneum, 1971.	Preschool
Where the Lilies Bloom, V. & B. Cleaver, New York, Lippincott, 1970.	Secondary

Reference Booklets

"Answers to a Child's Questions About Death," Peter Stellman, Guideline Publishers, Stamford, NY 12167. No price available. The booklet contains sketches, questions and answers designed to be read with children.

"Butterflies, Grandpa, and Me," Bruce Conley, Thum Printing, 116 W. Pierce St., Elburn, IL 60119 (312) 365-6415. $2.10 per copy.

"Children and Death," Alan Wolfelt, OGR Service Corporation, Box 3586, Springfield, IL 62708. No price available.

"Children Die, Too," Joy Johnson and Dr. S.M. Johnson, Centering Corporation, Box 878, Council Bluffs, IA 51502. No price available. For parents who have experienced the death of a child.

"Crisis in the Family," Vivian Cadden, National Research Bureau Inc., Chicago, IL. No price available. Emphasizes how friends and relatives can help a family experiencing a crisis.

"Death; What Do You Say to a Child?" Glen Davidson, OGR Service Corporation, Box 3586, Springfield, IL 62708. No price available.

"Do You Want to Help Me? The Art of Relating," Stephen R. Henderson, Full Circle Counseling Inc., Box 2726, Staunton, VA 24401. $1.75 per copy. For volunteers, relatives and professionals.

"For People Who Hurt . . . When Someone Dies," Bruce Conley and Karen Howard, Thumb Printing, Creative Marketing, PO 2423, Springfield, IL 62705. No price available. Poems pertaining to the death of infants, expressing feelings people have associated with grief and death.

"The Grief of Parents When a Child Dies," Margaret Miles, The Compassionate Friends Headquarters, P.O. Box 1347, Oakbrook, IL 60521. $1.25 in bulk; $1.75 per copy. The many facets of parental and sibling grief are discussed in a clear and sensitive manner.

"Handling the Holidays," Bruce Conley, Thum Printing, 116 W. Pierce St., Elburn, IL 60119, (312) 365-6415. No price available.

"Healing Grief," Amy Hillyard Jensen, Medic Publishing Company, Box O, Issaquah, WA 98027. $1.00 plus 50¢ postage for handling; bulk rate for 10 or more booklets.

"Helping Your Grieving Friend," The Center for Grief Counseling and Education, Inc., Box 1377, Madison, WI 57301. 25¢ per copy. Gives specific suggestions for friends and relatives of the bereaved.

"Is There Anything I Can Do To Help?" Amy Hillyard Jensen, Medic Publishing Company, Box O, Issaquah, WA 98027. $1.25 for 5 copies, bulk rate for 10 or more copies. Twenty suggestions for friends and relatives of grieving survivors.

"Overcoming Your Grief," Donald W. Steele, Ph.D., The Center for Grief Counseling and Education Inc., Box 1377, Madison, WI 53701. $2.00 per copy, 75¢ up to 25 copies, additional bulk rates. A 14-page booklet containing practical suggestions for the grieving person.

"Rainbows After a Storm," Susan Erling, 1515 N. Dale Street, St. Paul, MN 55117. $5.00 per copy includes postage, bulk rate available. "Touching poetry on pregnancy, pregnancy loss, grief, adoption, prematurity and multiple births."

"Talking with Young Children About Death," Mrs. Rogers Neighborhood, Pittsburgh Family Communications, 4802 Fifth Avenue, Pittsburgh, PA 15213. 50¢ per copy.

"The Subsequent Child," Carolyn Szybist, RN, U.S. Department of Health, Education and Welfare, Public Health Service, Health Services Administration, Bureau of Community Health Services, Rockville, MA 20857. No price available.

"When Hello Means Goodbye," Pat Schwiebert, RN, and Paul Kirk, MD, University of Oregon Health Services Center, Department of Ob-Gyn, 3181 S. Sam Jackson Park Rd., Portland, Oregon 97201. $1.50 per copy (make checks payable to Ob-Gyn Professors.) A guide for parents whose child dies at birth or shortly after.

"When Your Baby Dies," Boulder County Hospice, Inc., 2118 14th St., Boulder, CO 80302. 50¢ each, 40¢ for 25, additional bulk rates. Answers questions which arise after the death of an infant, including seeing and holding the baby, final arrangements, your feelings and the hospital staff's feelings.

"Where's Jess?" Centering Corporation, PO Box 3367, Omaha, NE 68013-0367. $2.35 per copy, bulk rate available. A booklet for parents experiencing miscarriage, stillbirth or newborn death.

Audio-Visual

"Death of a Dream: When a Baby Dies," Distributor: Boulder County Hospice Inc., 218 14th Street, Boulder, CO 80302, 20 minutes. $94 to purchase, $30 for a two-week rental. Re-creates birth and death experiences in the hospital, with candid conversation among parents which provides information for professionals and friends about helping the parents.

"Death of a Newborn," "Discussions with Parents of a Malformed Baby," "Discussions with Parents of Premature Infants." Health Sciences Communications Center, Case Western Reserve University. Order from Polymorph Films, 118 South Street, Boston, MA 02111, (617) 542-2004.

"Death of a Wished-For Child," Distributor: OGR Service Corporation, P.O. Box 3586, Springfield, IL 62708. (With booklet, Understanding the Death of the Wished-For Child).

"Memories," Distributor: SHARE, St. Joseph's Hospital, 800 E. Carpenter St., Springfield, IL 62702. A video-cassette directed to professionals on how to be helpful after a miscarriage, stillbirth or a newborn death.

"To Pick Up the Pieces," Distributor: Twenty-Twenty Media, Springfield, IL 62708, (217) 753-2541, 37 minutes.

"To Touch Today," Distributor: Creative Marketing, P.O. Box 2432, Springfield, IL 62705 (also available in booklet form), (217) 528-1756.

"We Were Sad, Remember," from IFDA, 1045 Outer Park Drive, Suite 120, Springfield, IL 62704.

"Where is Dead?" from IFDA, 1045 Outer Park Drive, Suite 120, Springfield, IL 62704.

INDEX

INTRODUCING

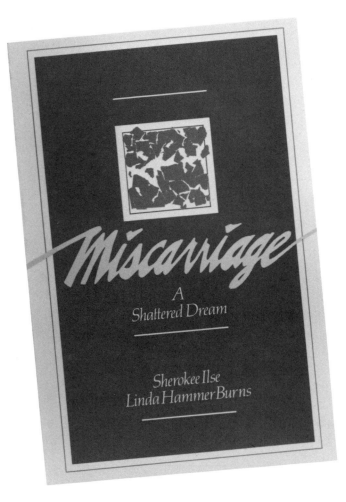

This new work is a welcome resource for those who have suffered a miscarriage as well as for their professional caregivers, family members, and friends. It offers a compelling and insightful perspective on miscarriage. Sherokee Ilse and Linda Hammer Burns write from both personal and professional experience. They offer sensitive discussions of such topics as: emotional responses, medical information and procedures, habitual miscarriage, coping skills, memorial suggestions, and a comprehensive guide. A most thorough and well written guide.

$5.50 per book, postage included
Bulk rate available

A NOTE
FROM THE
AUTHOR

I would like to hear your comments about the usefulness of this book, suggestions for improving it and/or your personal experiences. I also would like to know about groups or organizations who might want the book or more information about this topic.

Please write to:

Sherokee Ilse
P.O. Box 165
Long Lake, MN 55356